Transform in Seven:

The Enlightening Path to Rapid Weight Loss and Lifelong Wellness

By

Dr Albert M. Brose

Disclaimer page

Table of contents

Introduction

Greetings from a transformational adventure beyond everyday life. More than simply a book, Transform in Seven: The Enlightening Path to Rapid Weight Loss and Lifelong Wellness, is a journey partner that will help you become a better, happier version of yourself. This journey will alter your perspective, transform your physical form, and revitalise your soul. You'll learn as you read these pages that losing weight is an emotional and spiritual awakening as much as a physical change. You'll discover how to feed your body with what it really needs, move it with pleasure and purpose, and pay attention to your body's whispers before they become screams. This book is your roadmap to navigating the maze of false information and shortcuts to long-term transformation.

Feed Your Mind, Body, and Spirit. We start by establishing the fundamentals of knowledge and comprehending the complex dance between well-being and diet. You'll learn about the components of a healthy diet and the significant advantages of mindful eating. Every mouthful and decision you make moves you closer to being a more enlightened person. You'll come face to face with the psychological obstacles that have been impeding your success as you go deeper. You'll discover how to use your mind's power to overcome challenges and turn them into opportunities. You'll feel more in control and aware of your inner strength with every chapter.

The Path to Enduring Well-Being. This book is your road map to a fuller life, not simply a trimmer physique. It's about finding health in a world of sickness, harmony in the midst of confusion, and serenity amid the storm. Not only will your body have changed by the time you read the last chapter, but you will have kindled a wellness fire that will burn brightly for the rest of your life. Your Metamorphosis Starts Here. Thus, in Seven, open your heart, take a deep breath, and be ready to Transform. Knowing the essence of who you are and the food that sustains it is the first step. Together, let's flip the page and go on this transforming journey.

Chapter 1: Being Aware of Change

There is a special place where purpose and change come together in the stillness before morning. Transform in Seven: The Enlightening Path to Rapid Weight Loss and Lifelong Wellness starts here, in this sacred hour. This book is a lighthouse leading you to the enlightened road of change, not just a collection of pages. Every adventure begins with a single step a choice that moves you from inaction to movement. This book is a testimony to the power of making an educated decision, so keep that in mind when you stand on the brink of change. It is a wake-up call for those who want to live a life full of energy and purpose rather than merely lose weight. The Harmony of Emotion and Science. This book is a beautiful synthesis of human experience and empirical data, a symphony of science and spirit. The most recent findings in nutrition and physiology research will be presented to you, along with gripping tales from people who have been there before you. The colourful tapestry of life that each chapter presents will amuse you and teach you useful techniques that will become the instruments of your metamorphosis.

Let us present you to David, whose struggle with the scale became a spiritual victory, and Anna, whose weight loss journey became a search for wholeness. Their tales are more than simply stories, they serve as mirrors, revealing your own potential. You are not alone when you go out on this trip, either. Respected medical experts support the tactics in front of you and stand by you. 'Transform in Seven' takes a novel method. It's more important to create a sustainable lifestyle than it is to simply lose weight, holistic health pioneer Dr. Michael Richardson asserts. The Start of Your Adventure. The first phase of your metamorphosis begins to take shape when the first rays of dawn appear in the sky. It's time to accept the enlightened road that lies ahead and wake up to change. You will get closer to the person you are intended to be with every page you turn. Get ready to flip the page because you are about to enter a world where wellness is attainable, transformation is conceivable, and your path to long-term health starts. Now that you have this base, you may go on to the next phase of your journey toward enlightenment and change, where the building blocks of nourishment are waiting for you.

1.1 The Choice to Change

The route to change starts with a choice, just as a thousand miles start with a single step. You are now faced with a choice between living the life you want and living the one you now do. This is the moment of commitment. There is always a trigger for change a revelation that makes the need for change obvious. Some people believe that the picture depicts the reality. To others, it's the sincere counsel of a physician. We examine these crucial times in this chapter from the perspective of those who have dealt with them head-on. Accepting the Challenge. Making the daring decision to change is admirable. It's a proclamation that you're prepared to take charge and an acknowledgment that the current situation is untenable. Here, we explore the emotional process that goes along with choosing to make a change, facing our anxieties, and strengthening our determination.

The Ability to Choose, Your choice to change is a profound declaration of your potential and self-worth. Making the decision to put your health and well-being first comes with choices. Knowing that this subchapter is the first step toward a significant and long-lasting transformation will empower you. Meet James, who completed his first marathon and lost over 100 pounds as a result of his transformational choice. His narrative serves as a tribute to the ability of one choice to drastically change the trajectory of a life. A well-known nutritionist named Dr. Angela Martinez asserts that deciding to transform is the most important step towards attaining wellness. It's the foundation upon which all successful weight loss journeys are built. You'll flip a new page and take with you the knowledge that choosing to shift signifies both the end of old behaviours and the start of a new, enlightened route to healing. Building on this basis, the next subchapter, Understanding Your Body, will provide insights into the body that you use to navigate life's path.

1.2 Recognizing Your Body

Understanding our body, the vehicle that takes us through life is a prerequisite for transformation. This chapter takes you on a thorough exploration of the amazing, intricate human anatomy, That sustains us, empowers us, and, when understood, can be the greatest ally in our journey to wellness. Your body is more than flesh and bone, it is a symphony of processes, a masterpiece of biological engineering. Here, we unravel the mysteries of metabolism, the nuances of nutrition, and the wonders of the body's own healing powers. This knowledge is not just power, it is the power to change.

The Narrative of Nutrition. We will explore the role of macronutrients and micronutrients, the impact of different foods on our bodies, and how to harness this knowledge for weight loss and health. This section is not about dieting; it's about making informed choices that nourish and sustain. Understanding your body is also a journey of self-discovery. It's about tuning in to the subtle signals your body sends and learning to interpret them. This subchapter will guide you through this process, teaching you to become fluent in the language of your own physiology.

Real Stories, Real Inspiration. Meet Sarah, whose understanding of her body's unique needs led her to not just lose weight but also to overcome a chronic health condition. Her story is a beacon for all who seek to transform, illustrating the profound impact of knowledge applied.

Endorsed by Experts. Knowing your body is the foundation of any successful health journey, says prominent integrative medicine physician Dr. Lucas Nguyen. This book supplies the understanding needed to make that trip successful.

As you end this subchapter, you take with you the idea that your body is not a barrier to conquer, but a collaborator in your change. The following subchapter, Setting Realistic Goals, will build upon this acquired information, helping you create a road to success in your quest for health.

1.3 Setting Realistic Goals

In the tapestry of change, each thread represents a goal delicately crafted, deliberate, and necessary. 1.3 Setting Realistic Goals is the section where dreams are distilled into practical goals, where ambitions meet the roadmap of reality. Goals are the milestones of development, the lighthouses that lead us through the veil of uncertainty. Here, we go into the art of defining objectives that are not only desired but feasible.

This subchapter will teach you to blend ambition with pragmatism, ensuring that your path is defined with feasible wins. To sail the path ahead, you must build a compass of clear goals, quantifiable, and time-bound. This section will provide you with the tools to create a personalized blueprint for success, one that resonates with your unique journey and aligns with your deepest values.

Meet Michael, whose simple aim of walking a mile a day evolved into a marathon. His tale is a tribute to the power of realistic goal setting a narrative that will encourage you to take the steps, however little, towards your own victory.

Endorsed by Wisdom. Setting realistic goals is the bedrock of sustainable weight loss, emphasizes Dr. Emily Tran, a recognized voice in behavioral health. This book offers a pragmatic approach to goal setting that can lead to real change. As you flip the page, remember that each goal is a promise to yourself a promise of dedication, effort, and development. The next subchapter, Preparing for the Journey, will build on this foundation, providing you with the tools you need to go on this life-changing adventure.

1.4 Planning for the Journey

As we stand on the verge of transformation, 1.4 Preparing for the Journey is the subchapter that will provide you with the fundamentals for the transforming journey ahead. It's about setting the basis for success, making sure that every step is sturdy and confident. Preparation serves as the foundation for the transformational edifice. This part focuses on the practical components of preparedness, such as arranging your surroundings, preparing your nourishment, and aligning your thinking with your objectives. It is about establishing an environment that promotes change, both inside and outside.

Strategy for Preparation. Here, we offer a methodical approach to preparation, from diet planning to exercise scheduling. You'll learn how to foresee obstacles and prepare backup strategies. This section serves as your tactical guidance for converting intentions into actions. Learn about Emma, who changed her life by precisely organizing her weight reduction journey, and Carlos, whose thorough preparation helped him overcome years of harmful behaviors.

endorsements of efficacy. Preparation is a critical component of any successful health initiative, according to Dr. Rebecca Sun, a renowned wellness coach. The strategies in 'Transform in Seven' are a blueprint for effective preparation. As you finish this subchapter, you have the certainty that you are prepared to go on this trip. The next chapter awaits, in which the dietary pillars will strengthen your road to quick weight reduction and long-term well-being. Let the journey begin.

Chapter 2: Nutritional Fundamentals

Nutrition is important to the complicated dance of health and well-being. It's more than just counting calories or following fad diets, it's about understanding the alchemy that takes place within your body when you decide what to eat. Welcome to the heart of your transformation: the realm of nutritional fundamentals.

1. Science of Eating, Nutrition is more than just a plate of food it's a symphony of molecules that control life. Let's look into the science of macronutrients (carbohydrates, proteins, and fats) and micronutrients (vitamins and minerals). Each nutrient has a specific role in your body, ranging from providing energy to supporting cellular functions. Remember, your body is a finely tuned machine, and the fuel you choose matters.

2. Maintaining a Balanced Diet is essential for long-term wellness. We'll talk about how to create a balanced diet that nourishes your body while also satisfying your taste buds. Learn about portion control, food groups, and the

practice of mindful eating. Discover the joy of colorful fruits, leafy vegetables, and whole grains. Your plate is a canvas, let us paint it with health.

3. Water is essential for health and hydration. Dehydration can undermine your weight-loss efforts and impair cognitive function. We'll delve into the importance of staying hydrated, the signs of thirst (often masked as hunger), and practical tips to ensure you're sipping your way to vitality. Remember, your body is 60% water; honor this elemental connection.

4. The Role of Supplements, Supplements are like sidekicks they enhance your journey but can't replace the hero (whole foods). We'll demystify vitamins, minerals, and herbal supplements. When should you consider supplementation Which ones are supported by science And when is actual food the best choice Let's explore this supplement labyrinth together.

Success Stories, Meet Lisa, who corrected her prediabetes with focused dietary choices, and Mark, whose joint discomfort disappeared when he adopted an anti-inflammatory diet. Their tales show the transformational impact of food.

Expert Insights, Understanding your body is the cornerstone of health, emphasized by Dr. Maya Patel, a renowned dietician. It's not about restriction it's about nourishment.

As you end this chapter, remember that every mouthful you eat is a vote for your well-being. The next chapter, The science of Eating, awaits a voyage into the mind-body link that will further deepen your transformation. Your body is a temple, and the food you pick is the holy sacrifice. Let's nurture it with purpose.

2.1 The Science of Eating

Welcome to the fascinating realm of nutritional science, where each meal is a complicated interaction of chemistry and biology that sustains our basic survival. In 2.1 The Science of Eating, we dig into the molecular magic that keeps us going, examining how the decisions we make at the table impact every facet of our existence.

Understanding Macronutrients. Our bodies are wonderful machines that need the correct nutrition to flourish. We'll look at the science behind macronutrients, which are the proteins, carbs, and fats that make up our diet. Proteins are the fundamental building blocks of life, responsible for tissue healing and enzyme production. Carbohydrates are the fundamental source of energy, propelling all actions, from idea to step. Fats are essential for hormonal synthesis and food absorption. They compose the trinity of nutrients that promote our health.

The role of micronutrients, While macronutrients may take the stage, micronutrients play an important supporting role. Vitamins and minerals, although required in lower amounts, are important for good health. They defend our bodies from illness, promote development, and maintain the appropriate functioning of body systems. In this part, we'll study the 'invisible' nutrients that create a noticeable influence on our well-being. The metabolic process is the motor that drives all living things. Our bodies turn the food we eat into energy via this process. To shed pounds and feel more energized, we'll take a look at this complex system and see how it works. To find out how to effectively control your weight, you need to know your metabolism.

Real-Life Transformations: A Case Study of Alex, a man who lost weight and gained muscle by studying the science of nutrition, is our hero. Priya is another example, she went from prediabetic to normal after focusing on nutritional science. Their tales are not merely inspirational they are evidence of the power of education.

Endorsements from Experts, Understanding the science of eating is transformational, explains renowned nutritionist Dr. Helen Cho. This book explains the principles in an understandable and practical manner.

What you put into your body is more than simply fuel for your transformation. when you flip the page, you take this understanding with you. Balancing Your Diet, the next subchapter, will expand on this idea and show you how to include healthy food in your weight reduction plan. Let's go on this adventure of discovery together, where science meets sustenance, and every meal is a step towards a better you.

2.2 Macronutrients and Micronutrients

In the complicated ballet of nutrition, macronutrients and micronutrients take center stage. These are the building elements of vitality the letters that construct the language of health.

Let's study their responsibilities, comprehend their importance, and learn how to use them for our well-being.

1. Macronutrients: The Energy Providers

Carbohydrates: These are the body's principal source of energy. From the modest oatmeal to the sophisticated quinoa, carbs nourish our muscles, energize our minds, and keep us going. But not all carbohydrates are equal; some produce fast bursts of energy (simple sugars), while others maintain us over the long term (complex carbs).

Proteins: Think of proteins as the building workers of your body. They heal tissues, create enzymes, and comprise the backbone of muscles. Amino acids the Lego blocks of proteins are important for development and repair. Include lean meats, beans, and dairy in your diet to satisfy your protein demands.

Fats: Fats have been wrongly maligned, yet they're important for wellness. They insulate our organs, stabilize cell membranes, and function as messengers inside our bodies. Opt for healthy fats like avocados, almonds, and olive oil.

Remember, fat isn't the enemy it's a buddy in moderation.

2. Micronutrients: The Silent Heroes

Vitamins: These are the superheroes of our immune system, eyesight, and general health. From vitamin C (the defender against colds) to vitamin D (the sunshine vitamin), each serves a particular function. Fruits, vegetables, and fortified meals are excellent sources.

Minerals: These are the unsung heroes who keep our bones healthy, our neurons firing, and our hearts pumping. Calcium, magnesium, and iron, They're the minerals that matter. Leafy greens, nuts, and whole grains are mineral-rich companions.

3. The Balance Equation Like a symphony, our bodies thrive on harmony. Balancing macronutrients and micronutrients is crucial. Too much or too little of any nutrient might disturb the symphony. Aim for a variety of colors, textures, and tastes. Your plate should resemble a rainbow, not a monochromatic one.

4. Real-Life Transformations Meet Rachel, who restored her weariness by altering her

macronutrient ratios, and Jake, whose micronutrient-rich diet improved his skin health. Their experiences remind us that nutrition isn't theoretical it's practical magic.

5. Expert Insights, Understanding macronutrients and micronutrients empowers you to make informed choices, says Dr. Emily Chen, a noted nutritionist. It's not about counting calories it's about nourishing your body.

As you close this section, remember that every mouthful you consume is an investment in your health. The following subchapter, Balancing Your Diet, awaits a voyage into the art of making meals that connect with your body's demands.

2.3 Balancing Your Diet

In the delicate dance of nutrition, balance is the choreography that keeps us in tune. Imagine your plate as a seesaw one side filled with nutrition, the other with flavor and enjoyment. Balancing your food isn't about restriction it's about creating a symphony of tastes that feed both body and spirit.

1. The Art of Portion Control Like a conductor holding a baton, you have the capacity to arrange your meals. Portion management is the rhythm that guarantees you don't overwhelm the stage. Consider your plate split it into parts. Fill half with colourful vegetables the virtuosos of vitamins and fiber. Reserve a quarter for lean proteins the maestros of muscle regeneration. The remaining quarter Whole grains or starchy vegetables the harmonious carbohydrates that power your day.

2. Quality Above Quantity There are differences in the composition of calories. A hundred calories of broccoli dance differently in your body than a hundred calories of cookies. Choose nutrient-dense foods the soloists that offer vitamins, minerals, and antioxidants. Opt for nutritious grains, lean proteins, and healthy fats. These virtuosos not only quench your appetite but also fuel your cells.

3. The Flavor Palette Imagine your taste receptors as painters, desiring a canvas of diversity. Spices, herbs, and seasonings bring colour to your food. Turmeric gives warmth basil, freshness cinnamon, depth. Experiment with flavors the acidity of citrus, the umami of

mushrooms, the sweetness of roasted peppers. Your plate becomes a gallery of taste.

4. Mindful Eating Slow down. Savor each mouthful. Mindful eating isn't simply about what you eat it's about how you eat. Put away distractions, the screens, the tension. Engage your senses. Notice the crispness of an apple and the smoothness of yogurt. Listen to your body's signals. Are you full Are you satisfied Mindful eating turns meals into moments of presence.

5. Real-Life Transformations Meet Sarah, who balanced her diet by introducing colourful salads and lean meats. And there's David, who found the pleasure of portion management and dropped weight without feeling deprived. Their experiences remind us that balancing isn't a tightrope it's a dance floor.

6. Expert Insights, Balancing your diet is about nourishing your body while honouring your cravings, explains Dr. Elena Rodriguez, a noted nutritionist. It's not about restriction it's about equilibrium.

As you end this subchapter, remember that your plate is a canvas a masterpiece ready to be painted with health. The following subchapter,

Hydration and Health, awaits a trip into the elixir of life that will further satisfy your desire for well-being. Balance isn't a tightrope it's a dance floor where health and enjoyment waltz together.

2.4 Hydration and Health

Water The elixir of life. It rushes through our veins, fueling every cell, whispering secrets of life. In this subchapter, we plunge into the crystal-clear depths of hydration, studying its enormous influence on our well-being.

1. The Thirsty Truth

Imagine your body as a sensitive ecology. Water is its currency, moving through rivers of blood, washing organs, and cooling the flames of metabolism. When you're dehydrated, this ecosystem falters. Your vitality wanes, your skin loses its sheen, and even your thoughts become dry. Listen to your body's whisper those tiny indications that indicate, I need water.

2. Beyond the Eight Glasses Myth

The eight glasses a day guideline is a well-intentioned fiction. In actuality, your hydration demands are as unique as your fingerprint. Factors including environment, exercise level, and individual variances play a symphony of thirst. So, how much water do you need Pay heed to your body's messages. When your mouth feels dry, when your pee is amber instead of light gold, it's time to sip.

3. The Weight Loss Connection

Hydration and weight reduction are dancing partners. When you're well-hydrated, your metabolism pirouettes beautifully. Water cranks up the calorie-burning motors, making weight reduction more efficient. Plus, sometimes thirst masquerades as hunger. Before reaching for that food, ask yourself, Am I really hungry, or just thirsty

4. The Skin's Quench

Your skin the canvas of your wellness. When you're hydrated, it sparkles like morning dew on a flower. Deprive it, and it crinkles like dry soil. Hydration plumps your skin, minimizes wrinkles, and gives you that radiant appeal. Forget pricey lotions; water is your finest beauty secret.

Real-Life Transformations

Meet Emily, who replaced her afternoon Coke with a glass of water and saw her energy soar. And there's Jake, who kept a water bottle by his side and dropped weight without feeling deprived. Their experiences remind us that change frequently starts with a mere drink.

Expert Insights, Hydration is the cornerstone of health, says Dr. Maria Rodriguez, a noted nutritionist. It's not just about drinking water it's about honoring your body's need for balance.

As you end this subchapter, remember that every drop counts. The next chapter, The Psychology of Eating, awaits a voyage inside the mind's wants and desires. Let's drink to health, one glass at a time. Your body sings a liquid symphony listen intently, and it will lead you to well-being.

Chapter 3: The Psychology of Eating

Embark on a transforming journey into the fascinating fabric of our connection with food. This chapter goes deep into the psychological foundations that impact our eating habits, unraveling the threads of emotion, cognition, and habit that weave the fabric of our dietary patterns. As we explore the complexity of desire and satisfaction, we reveal the subtle but strong forces that shape our choices, create our habits, and ultimately influence our relationship with the very food that gives us life. We examine the quiet exchanges between the mind and the body, the silent talks at the dinner table, and the quiet contemplations inside the sanctuary of the kitchen.

Here, we lay bare the emotional links that bind us to our meals, the cultural tapestries that define our palates, and the personal tales that tell the story of every mouthful. We face the specters of stress eating and the solace found in the familiar scents of nostalgia, seeking knowledge and control over the urges that lead us wrong.

This chapter is not only a compilation of facts and instructions it is an invitation to a more conscious communion with our meals. It is a cry to arms against the mindless chewing and a roadmap for a more conscious, more harmonious living with the food that nourishes our very being.

As we shut the pages of this chapter, we do not leave behind a trail of rigorous rules or inflexible diet programs. Instead, we carry forward a fresh insight a wisdom that allows us to make choices that resonate with our innermost selves, decisions that value our health and well-being. With each turn of the page, we get closer to a future where food is not an opponent but an ally a participant in the dance of life, a co-creator of our destiny. As we transit easily into the next chapter, we take with us the lessons learned, ready to apply them to the domain of fitness and movement, where the symphony of nutrition harmonizes with the melody of motion.

3.1 Emotional Eating and Awareness

Nourishing the Soul: Beyond Calories and Cravings

In the quiet corners of our kitchens, where the hum of the refrigerator meets the murmurs of our emotions, emotional eating takes center stage. It's a covert affair an intimate dance between our emotions and our plates.

The Midnight Fridge Chronicles

Picture this: a moonlight kitchen, its linoleum floor cold against bare feet. The clock nudges beyond midnight, as the world outside slumbers. Yet, behind these confines, a lone individual stands drawn by more than hunger. The refrigerator door creaks open, displaying a scene of comfort leftover lasagna, a half-eaten chocolate bar, and a container of vanilla ice cream. Emotional eating, two words that capture a world of human experience. It's not about nourishment it's about consolation. When life's problems weigh heavy, we seek shelter in the comforting embrace of food. The warmth of a piece of apple pie mimics the warmth of a mother's love. The crunch of potato chips drowns out the chorus of worry.

The Whispers of Cravings

But what are we genuinely feeding Our bodies or our souls The border fades when we reach for that second cookie, the one that tastes like reminiscence and forgiveness. We've all been there, the breakup pint of ice cream, the celebration cake slice, the stress-induced bag of pretzels. These desires mimic our emotions, and our plates become canvases for unsaid sensations. Awareness is our light in this maze. It's the pause before the first bite, the investigation into our hunger's genesis. Are we actually hungry, or are we seeking solace When joy, grief, or tension tempt us into the pantry, we must ask What am I truly hungry for

The Dance of Mind and Mouth.

Emotional eating isn't a villain; it's a messenger. It whispers truths our conscious brains frequently disregard. Perhaps the chocolate bar recalls memories of childhood birthdays. Maybe the salty popcorn softens the agony of loneliness. Our aim is not to avoid emotional eating but to know its signs. Pause, Breathe and Reflect, In this dance, we learn to discern between bodily hunger and emotional hunger. We respect both the grumble of an empty stomach and the sorrow of a tired heart. We pick consciously, recognizing that sometimes a salad feeds more than just our cells, and sometimes a warm cup of soup cures more than a cold.

And so, as we finish this chapter, let us take this understanding forward. Let us step cautiously in our kitchens, listening to the whispers of our appetites. Emotional eating need not be our opponent it may be our ally a compass directing us toward self-compassion, a connection between our hearts and our plates.

In the next sub chapter we will learn about Breaking Bad Habits, How we can demolish the habits that no longer benefit us and clear the way for mindful nutrition. May your trip through these pages be as nutritious as the meals you pick.

3.2 Breaking Bad Habits

Rewiring Our Relationship with Food.

Habits, the unseen builders of our lives. They shape our mornings, our mealtimes, and our nocturnal desires. Some behaviors urge us toward health while others, like subtle saboteurs, lead us away.

The Familiar Grooves

Picture this: the workplace breakroom, a fluorescent-lit sanctuary of vending machines and shared munchies. It's 3 p.m., and the siren song of the candy bar calls. You've been here before the mid-afternoon slump, the desire for a fast pick-me-up. Your hand extends out, almost automatically. But wait. Pause and Breathe. Breaking harmful behaviors involves more than willpower it demands deliberate intervention. Imagine a red stop sign in your mind the instant you reach for that bag of chips, STOP. Reflect. Is this habit benefitting me Or is it a well-worn groove moving away from my health goals.

The Rituals We Keep

Our brains thrive on routines. They seek solace in the familiar, the usual morning cereal, the routine commute to work, the night time dessert. But what if we rewrote these scripts What if we replaced the midnight cookie raid with a relaxing cup of herbal tea What if our morning habit comprised stretching instead of perusing through social media. Awareness is our compass. It steers us away from autopilot and toward deliberate decisions. As we drink that morning coffee, we ask: Is this a habit or a conscious act We analyze our routines, studying their roots. Perhaps that daily chocolate square ties back to childhood incentives. Perhaps the late-night munching mimics our parents' behaviors.

The Power of Substitution

Breaking poor behaviors isn't about restriction it's about replacement. When the need for sweet treats arises, we go for a handful of almonds or a crisp apple. We replace thoughtless chewing with focused enjoyment. We swap the shame of empty calories for the delight of wholesome choices. Small steps, we tell ourselves. The elevator becomes the steps. The soda becomes sparkling water. The late-night TV binge becomes a chapter in an excellent novel. Each decision is a brick along the road toward change.

And so, as we finish this subchapter, let us respect our habits the old and the new. Let us celebrate the victories the foregone dessert, the additional glass of water milestones on our path. Overcoming unhealthy habits isn't a war it's a dance, a rhythm of purpose, a melody of transformation.

Next up is Chapter 3.3 Mindful Eating Strategies where we relish each mouthful, bringing the senses to the table. May your habits be partners, helping you toward lifetime well-being.

3.3 Mindful Eating Strategies

Savoring Each Morsel: A Symphony of the Senses

In the silent drama of our dining rooms, where forks meet plates and tastes dance on taste senses, mindful eating takes center stage. It's not just about what we eat it's about how we consume.

The Art of Present Nourishment

Picture this: a sun-kissed morning, a dish of fresh berries before you. The strawberries flaunt their seeds like little stars, the blueberries explode with azure promise. You raise the spoon, but before it hits your lips, you halt. Breathe. You're not only eating you're savoring a purposeful act of presence. Mindful eating urges us to be totally involved with our meals. It's not about gulping down lunch at our offices or devouring supper while looking through social media. No, it's an homage to the senses. As you raise your fork, observe the colors the scarlet of a tomato, the jade of spinach. Feel the textures the crunch of almonds, the silkiness of avocado. Inhale the aromas the warmth of cinnamon, the earthiness of roasted veggies.

The Symphony of Chew

Chew carefully. Let tastes unfold. Each mouthful is a note in the symphony of nutrition. As you chew, enzymes dance, breaking down food into its essential melodies carbohydrates, proteins, and lipids. The more we chew, the more we extract. It's not only about digestion it's about absorption of nutrients, sure, but also of life's moments. Distractions are the saboteurs of mindful eating. Put away the electronics let the meal be your whole attention. In this silent connection with food, we nurture not just our bodies but also our spirits. We taste the sunshine that caressed the tomatoes, and the rain that swelled the grains of rice. We respect the effort of farmers, the craft of cooks, and the wonder of development.

The Fullness of Enough

Mindful eating isn't about limitation it's about abundance. It's about recognizing when the body says, I've had enough. It's the moment you push the plate away, not out of denial but out of respect. It's the realization that fullness isn't a finish line it's a gentle curves place where hunger meets contentment.

As we close this subchapter, let us carry this mindfulness beyond the table. Let us savor not only flavors but also moments the laughter shared over a meal, the quiet joy of a perfectly ripe peach. For mindful eating isn't a diet it's a celebration feast of awareness, a banquet of gratitude.

Next up is Chapter 3.4 The Power of Positive Thinking where we season our plates with hope and flavor our lives with possibility. May dinners become magical with your forks acting as wands.

3.4 The Positive Thought Process

Developing Inward Nutrition, Thought seeds sprout in the garden of our brains. Some become bright blossoms, some become gnarly weeds. Our mental state is just as important to weight reduction as the foods we choose.

The Relationship Between the Mind and Body. Imagine someone standing in front of a mirror and evaluating their image. The gaze skims across arcs, flaws, and ambitions. However, what if we turned our attention inward What if we could see the ideas that shape the physical body as well

Being positive is a conscious decision, not just hope. It's the conviction that change is possible and that each step we take to improve our health is like painting a new picture of our lives. This is confirmed by scientific studies, our bodies react when we see achievement. Cells dance, hormones change, and metabolic pathways wake up.

Case Studies on Victory

Introducing Sarah, a teacher who struggled with obesity for many years. A storm of self-doubt raced through her mind: I've tried every diet. I will never alter. But later, she came across a book that was somewhat similar to this one. She had read about the benefits of visualization and the strength of affirmations. Sarah's daily motto was, I am becoming healthier. Her routines gradually changed. She preferred stairs to elevators and salads to fries. Not only did the pounds melt, but her incredulity did too. And there's Mark, a middle-aged businessman struggling with weight gain brought on by stress. His days were a haze of missed meals and deadlines. Mark discovered, however, that stress had a bodily cost in addition to a mental one. The stress hormone cortisol stuck to his waist. Armed with information, he adopted mindfulness practices including taking deep breaths during meetings, going for walks in the park, and having moments of appreciation. He lost weight steadily, but not quickly. His stress level dropped along with his waistline.

The Opinion of Medical Experts. According to well-known nutritionist Dr. Elena Rodriguez, Positive thinking isn't a placebo. It acts as a trigger. Patients stick to healthy behaviors when they have confidence in their abilities to change. Their bodies react; inflammation decreases and metabolism speeds up.

Psychotherapist Dr. James Harper agrees: Our ideas influence our actions. Visualizing achievement causes our brains to develop pathways geared toward it. It's called neuroplasticity, the brain's capacity to reorganize itself, not magic.

As we wrap up this chapter, let's remember to take care of our thoughts as well as our bodies. The phrase I can't should be changed to I am becoming. Let's commemorate each salad and every dessert passed over as turning points in our journey. Because thinking positively is a habit that we leave behind for ourselves and future generations, rather than a passing feeling.

In the next chapter we will learn about Fitness and Movement, where we investigate the tango between resilience and perspiration by putting on our shoes. May the architects of your change be your ideas.

Chapter 4: Movability and Strength

The brilliant colors of life and vigor are intertwined with the threads of fitness and movement in the great tapestry of well-being. This chapter honors the body's amazing capacity for change brought about by physical exercise. It's a tribute to the perseverance and sweat that clear the way to a better version of yourself. As we set out on our adventure, we explore the significant effects that exercise has on our health. We examine the science behind exercise and how it contributes to improving life quality as well as helping people lose weight. We reveal the tales of people who have danced with their shadows and come out into the light of health, those who have used their own bodies as a tool to forge a path toward well-being.

We'll rely on the knowledge of medical experts who promote incorporating exercise into our everyday lives as a valued component of our schedule rather than as a duty. Their voices resound over the pages, providing direction and consolation as they impart knowledge on how movement may serve as a catalyst for transformation. This chapter focuses on developing a respectful and admiring connection with our bodies rather than merely providing workouts to help us lose weight. It's about appreciating the power of lifting weights, the elegance of a yoga position, or the rhythm of an early morning jog. Finding the kinds of movement that speak to our souls, bring us alive, and help us connect to our true selves is the goal.

We see the transformational effect of perseverance and determination via case studies. We might take inspiration from individuals who have overcome inertia and accepted the dynamic nature of fitness. Their achievements shine a light on the route for others to follow, acting as inspirational and uplifting beacons. Turning the pages serves as a reminder that exercise is a celebration of what our bodies are capable of, not a penalty for the foods we consume. We are urged to see exercise as a lifetime partner on our path to health rather than as a passing fad.

As this chapter comes to an end, we are really only getting started. We are starting a new chapter in our lives where physical activity and fitness aren't simply something we do they're essential components of who we are. The trip and the dance move on, guiding us into the next chapter where more sophisticated techniques are waiting to help us achieve our goals of well-being and health. I hope that your quest for fitness will be as fulfilling as the final goal and that you will always know that you are getting closer to being a better, healthier version of yourself.

4.1 The Effects of Exercise on Weight Loss

Weight reduction journeys sometimes begin with a glance in the mirror, but genuine change comes when we move away from our image and into activity. Exercise is the spark that fires the body's ability to reorganize itself, and this subchapter delves into the critical function it plays in weight reduction. When discussing weight loss, the narrative often centers on food. Exercise, on the other hand, ignites the way to long-term weight control. It's not just about how many calories you burn during a workout it's also about the after burn the heightened state of metabolism that continues to melt fat long after the sweat has dried.

The Science Behind Sweat

Scientific studies have repeatedly shown that regular physical exercise, paired with a well-balanced diet, is the most efficient strategy to lose and keep weight off. Exercise not only reduces fat deposits but also increases muscle mass, which burns more calories at rest than fat. This indicates that the more muscle you have, the more calories you burn, even if you don't exercise.

Success Stories: The Proof of the Pudding. Throughout this subchapter, we'll present inspiring stories about how people have used fitness to alter their bodies and lives. These examples, from the busy mom who made time for exercise to the office worker who switched his chair for a standing desk and a treadmill, are more than simply encouraging, they also demonstrate the power of movement.

Expert Insight: Words That Move Us

Exercise is promoted as a cornerstone of weight reduction by healthcare experts of all types, from nutritionists to personal trainers. Movement is medicine, they say, and the prescription is a regimen of daily exercise customized to your lifestyle. Whether it's a morning swim, an evening bike ride, or a midday stroll, the idea is to pick something you like and stick to it.

As we go through this subchapter, we'll present you with useful advice and activities to help you get started on your weight reduction journey. We'll talk about how to create realistic objectives, overcome mental hurdles to exercise and develop a long-term habit.

By the conclusion of 4.1 The Role of Exercise in Weight Loss, you'll not only grasp the how and why of exercise's influence on weight reduction, but you'll also feel ready and empowered to lace up your shoes and embark on a healthier, more active lifestyle.

Are you ready to flip the page Next, we'll look at 4.2 Overcoming Plateaus, in which we'll address the unavoidable hurdles on the path to health and identify ways to break through and move ahead. Let's begin active and alter not just our bodies, but also our brains and souls, on this health trip.

4.2 Planning Your Exercise Routine

In the pursuit of weight reduction, developing an exercise program is analogous to an artist creating a masterpiece. It's a personal path that takes patience, exploration, and a knowledge of one's own body. In this subchapter, we will look at how to create an exercise program that not only helps you lose weight but also becomes a sustainable and fun part of your daily routine. Personalization is key. Each person's body reacts differently to various types of exercise. What suits one person may not be appropriate for another. This is why customization is critical. We'll look at how to listen to your body's signals and customize your training routine to meet your own requirements, interests, and lifestyle.

Building a Foundation. We begin with the fundamentals establishing a foundation of regular physical exercise that may be expanded over time. This isn't about jumping headlong into a tough routine, but rather beginning at a rate that seems reasonable and progressively increasing intensity as your fitness increases.

Variety: The Spice of Life. To keep both the mind and body engaged, we bring diversity into the program. This might entail rotating between cardio, weight training, flexibility exercises, and other activities like yoga or sports. Variety not only reduces boredom but also challenges various muscle groups and promotes overall fitness.Setting Achievable Goals, Goal setting is a great motivator. We explore how to develop realistic, attainable objectives that bring direction and purpose to your fitness regimen. Whether it's jogging a particular distance, lifting a specified weight, or just committing to a number of exercises each week, defining objectives may keep you focused and on track.

The Role of Community. Often, the trip is made easier with companionship. We'll discuss the advantages of finding a workout companion, attending a fitness class, or being part of an online community. These ties may give support, accountability, and a feeling of camaraderie. Adaptation and Flexibility. Life is unpredictable, and so is the route to weight reduction. We'll examine how to adjust your fitness regimen to life's changes be it a hectic schedule, an injury, or a lack of drive. Flexibility in your approach helps you to remain committed even when circumstances vary.

As we wind up this subchapter, we prepare to transfer effortlessly into the next part of your fitness journey. With your individualized exercise program in hand, you're ready to tackle the obstacles ahead, including overcoming plateaus and customizing your workout for optimal efficacy. Coming up, we'll tackle 4.3 Overcoming Plateaus, where we'll learn to negotiate the unavoidable halt in progress and restart the momentum in your weight loss quest. Embark on this path with confidence, knowing that each step you take is a step towards a healthier, more vibrant self.

4.3 Overcoming Plateaus

In the terrain of weight reduction, plateaus are like mountains that challenge our determination, testing the strength of our dedication to fitness. This subchapter is devoted to conquering these apparently insurmountable difficulties, converting them into stepping stones toward our ultimate objective.

Understanding the Plateau. A weight reduction plateau happens when progress appears to cease despite keeping an exercise regimen and appropriate eating habits. It's a normal aspect of the body's adaptation process, as it grows more effective at completing familiar activities. Here, we'll look into the physiological components of plateaus and why they are a sign of development, not stagnation. Strategies to Break Through, We'll review numerous techniques to rekindle weight reduction, from changing nutritional intake to boosting exercises. Sometimes, the solution lies in modifying the kind of exercise, increasing the intensity, or even allowing for extra relaxation. We'll share practical ideas on how to listen to your body and alter your routine appropriately.

Success Stories: Climbing the Mountain. Through fascinating anecdotes, we'll discuss the experiences of others who've successfully conquered their plateaus. These anecdotes will not only amuse but also serve as a source of inspiration and learning, proving that with the appropriate approach, any plateau can be overcome.

Expert Advice: Scaling New Heights, Quotes and advice from fitness gurus and healthcare specialists will give other insights on navigating plateaus. Their views will reinforce the notion that plateaus are a natural part of the trip and can be conquered with patience and the appropriate mentality.

As we end this subchapter, we prepare to shift into the next part of your fitness journey. With fresh methods in hand and a renewed feeling of resolve, you're ready to confront any obstacle that comes your way. Up next, we'll move into 4.4 Rest and Recovery, where we'll learn the necessity of allowing our bodies the time they need to recover and get stronger. Embrace the plateau as a chance for progress, and let each step you take be a monument to your unshakable dedication to health and fitness.

4.4 Rest and Recovery

In the harmonic harmony of weight reduction and well-being, relaxation, and recuperation are the quiet beats that give the song its depth. This subchapter is an homage to the unsung heroes of transformation the quiet moments of healing that prepare the way for fresh energy and vitality.

The Silent Guardians of Progress. Rest and recuperation are not only interruptions in our program they are important components of a successful training approach. They enable our bodies to heal, renew, and strengthen after the exertions of exercise. Here, we'll investigate the science underpinning muscle healing and the body's incredible capacity to renew and adapt.

Case Studies: The Power of Pause. We'll present encouraging examples of folks who have achieved considerable weight reduction and credit a portion of their success to appropriate rest. These anecdotes will not only give significant insights but also act as emotional testaments to the importance of listening to one's body.

Scientific Backing: The Evidence of Ease. Referencing scientific research, we'll dig into how rest adds to metabolic efficiency, muscular development, and general wellness. These references will underline the value of including rest days in any training plan and how they may actually boost weight reduction efforts.

Expert Voices: The Chorus of Care. Quotes and testimonials from healthcare experts will reinforce the notion that rest is not laziness it's a type of self-care that is vital for long-term success. Rest is where the magic happens, they say, backing the tactics presented in this book for efficient weight reduction and recovery.

As we complete this subchapter, we prepare to move into the following chapter with a feeling of serenity and preparation. Understanding the function of rest and recuperation, you are now ready to approach your fitness path with a balanced viewpoint. In the forthcoming chapter, Advanced Weight Loss Strategies, we will examine creative approaches and strategies to further boost your path toward lifetime well-being. Embrace the healing power of rest and recuperation, and let it be the foundation upon which your fitness achievements are built.

Chapter 5: Advanced Weight Loss Strategies

In the path of transformation, Chapter 5 shines as a beacon of innovation, taking readers through the advanced tactics that pave the road to quick weight loss and lifetime well-being. This chapter offers a deep dive into the cutting-edge strategies that go beyond the fundamentals, presenting a fresh viewpoint on how to approach weight management with complexity and awareness. Here, we review the newest studies and approaches that have arisen on the subject of weight control. From the subtleties of metabolic fitness to the nuances of hormonal balance, this chapter illustrates the route for individuals who desire to perfect their approach to losing pounds.

Case Studies: Triumphs of Transformation. We provide fascinating case studies of people who have burst past boundaries utilizing these advanced tactics. Their experiences are not merely accounts of weight reduction but also testaments to the human spirit's potential for change and adaptation.

Scientific Validation: The Backbone of Innovation, Each strategy mentioned is supported by scientific research and respected sources, guaranteeing that you are obtaining knowledge that is not only new but also legitimate and dependable. This chapter doesn't simply tell, it proves the success of these tactics through the prism of evidence-based research.

Professional Endorsements: The Seal of Approval. Incorporating quotes and testimonials from healthcare professionals, this chapter provides an authoritative voice on the efficacy of the advanced strategies outlined. These endorsements serve as a powerful tool to persuade and reassure readers that they are on the right path.

As we conclude Chapter 5, we set the stage for the next chapter,The advanced strategies laid out here are not the end but a gateway to even greater understanding and success in weight management.

Looking ahead, Chapter 5.1 will build upon these foundations, focusing on Intermittent Fasting Demystified and how to sustain the remarkable progress made. Embark on this chapter with an open mind and a willing heart, ready to embrace Intermittent Fasting strategies that will transform your approach to weight loss and set you on a path to lifelong wellness.

5.1 Intermittent Fasting Demystified

Understanding Intermittent Fasting. Intermittent fasting (IF) is more than just a diet, it's an eating pattern that cycles between periods of fasting and eating. Instead of concentrating on particular meals, IF stresses when you should eat. Let's discuss the essential components of IF:

1. The Basics of IF Methods

16/8 Method (Leangains Protocol): This popular strategy incorporates a 8-hour eating window followed by a 16-hour fasting period. You may forgo breakfast or supper, depending on your taste.

Eat-Stop-Eat: For individuals familiar with fasting, this strategy requires a 24-hour fast once or twice a week.

5:2 Diet: On two nonconsecutive days each week, consume just 500–600 calories, while eating regularly on the other five days.

2. How IF Affects Your Body

When you fast, remarkable changes occur at the cellular and molecular levels:

Human Growth Hormone (HGH) Boost: HGH levels increase during fasting, promoting fat breakdown and muscle preservation.

Insulin Regulation: IF reduces insulin resistance, improving blood sugar control.

Cellular Repair: Fasting triggers essential cellular repair processes, enhancing overall health.

Gene Expression: Your body adjusts gene expression, optimizing metabolic pathways.

3. Weight Loss and Beyond

IF offers several benefits beyond weight loss:

Longevity: Animal studies link calorie restriction (similar to fasting) to longevity and reduced disease risk.

Brain Health: Fasting may enhance cognitive function and protect against neurodegenerative diseases.

Inflammation Reduction: Some research shows that IF decreases inflammation indicators.

As we end our investigation of IF, let's easily shift to the following section. Remember, this path toward wellness is about more than simply dropping poundsit's about adopting sustainable behaviors and lasting health. Stay tuned for the next chapter, when we dig into Understanding Metabolic Flexibility a critical piece of the jigsaw on your route to transformation!

5.2 Understanding Metabolic Flexibility

 The Dance of Energy: Fat and Carbs. Metabolic flexibility is like a delicate tango between your body's primary energy sources: fat and carbohydrates. Imagine your body as a skillful dancer, gracefully switching from one partner to another on the dance floor of metabolism.

1. The Metabolic Symphony

Fat-Burning Waltz: When you're metabolically flexible, your body twirls beautifully, burning fat for energy. During times of fasting or low-carb consumption, it pulls into stored fat stores. This dance keeps you slim and energetic.

Carb Cha-Cha: After a carb-rich meal, your body shifts gears. It cha-chas, using glucose from carbs. Excess glucose is stored as muscle glycogen, ready for your next energetic spin.

2. Insulin: The Choreographer, Insulin takes center stage in this metabolic ballet. Picture it as the choreographer, guiding the moves:

High Insulin Levels: In metabolically inflexible people, insulin is overzealous. It stimulates fat accumulation, leading to weight gain and health concerns.

Low Insulin Levels: Metabolically flexible dancers have well-timed insulin signals. Insulin rises, transfers glucose into muscle cells (as glycogen), and then elegantly quit the stage, enabling fat-burning to restart.

3. Cultivating Metabolic Flexibility

a. Diet Harmony

Entire Foods: Opt for entire, unprocessed foods. Minimize added sweets and refined carbohydrates. This harmonic diet decreases glucose and insulin levels, alleviating stress on your cells.

Intermittent Fasting: Take pauses from eating. Intermittent fasting facilitates the transition from sugar-burning to fat-burning. It's like giving your dancers a break before their next performance.

b. Exercise Rhythm

Daily Movement: Keep insulin nimble by being active. Dance, stroll, or stretch, it all counts. Your body enjoys a daily routine.

Strength Training: Build muscle. Muscles are insulin's favorite dancing partners they consume glucose effectively.

c. Restful Slumber

Sweet Dreams: Aim for 7 to 9 hours of excellent sleep. Sleep refreshes your dancers, ensuring they hit the appropriate steps throughout the day.

d. Stress-Free Pas de Deux

Stress Reduction: Stress disturbs the dancing. Practice mindfulness, deep breathing, or mild yoga. Your metabolic ballet flourishes in a tranquil setting.

As we end our investigation of metabolic flexibility, let's glide easily into the following subchapter: The Ketogenic Shift. Brace yourself for a daring journey into the realm of ketones and metabolic magic!

5.3 The Ketogenic Shift

Unlocking Metabolic Magic: The Keto Diet. The ketogenic diet often simply dubbed the keto diet is a potent tool for weight reduction and general health. Imagine it as a hidden path that takes your body away from carb-heavy highways and into the region of fat-burning bliss.

1. The Keto Symphony

Low Carb, High Fat: On the keto stage, carbohydrates take a backseat, while fats move into the forefront. By dramatically lowering carbohydrate consumption, your body switches gears. It's like driving off the freeway of glucose and taking a leisurely path through the region of ketones.

Ketosis Unleashed: In this metabolic state, your liver becomes an alchemist, changing stored fat into energy molecules. These ketones feed your brain, muscles, and organs. Say welcome to mental clarity and continuous vitality!

2. The Fat-Burning Ballet

Bye-Bye Insulin Spikes: The keto diet decreases insulin levels, which is excellent news for weight reduction. Insulin, our metabolic conductor, generally transfers glucose into cells. But on keto, it steps aside, enabling fat to take center stage.

Preserving Muscle, Losing Fat: Unlike crash diets, keto helps you burn fat while keeping crucial muscle mass. It's like molding your physique with precision.

3. The Keto Toolbox

a. Foods to Embrace

Healthy Fats: Avocados, nuts, seeds, and olive oil become your culinary buddies.

Protein in Moderation: Fish, poultry, and meat supply needed amino acids.

Leafy Greens: Spinach, kale, and other low-carb vegetables give color and nutrition.

b. Foods to Bid Adieu

Carb Farewell: Say farewell to wheat, rice, potatoes, and sweet delights.

Fruit Caution: Even fruits nature's candy take a backstage pass owing to their inherent sugars.

As we end our investigation of the keto diet, let's move gracefully into the following subchapter: Supplements and Weight Loss. Brace yourself for a tornado of information as we begin our transforming adventure!

5.4 Supplements and Weight Loss

Unlocking the Power of Supplements. Weight reduction supplements those small partners in our health journey often promise spectacular changes. But how can we discern reality from fiction Let's study the research, the tales, and the tactics that may genuinely increase your weight reduction journey.

1. The Science Behind Supplements

A Balanced Equation: Remember, supplements are not miracle bullets. They complement a healthy diet and an active lifestyle.

Evidence Matters: When contemplating supplements, depend on evidence-based research. Let's delve into some significant players:

a. Extract from Green Tea

The Metabolic Boost: Green tea extract contains catechins that may improve metabolism and fat oxidation.

Incidental Achievement: Meet Sarah, a dedicated educator. She lost weight gradually after starting to drink green tea every day. Science validated her claims.

b. Fatty Acids Omega-3

Heart-Healthy Allies: By lowering inflammation and enhancing insulin sensitivity, omega-3s promote heart health and may help with weight reduction.

Inspiring Adventure: John, a former fireman, increased the amount of omega-3 fish in his diet. His energy level increased and his waistline shrank.

2. Case Studies: Actual Individuals, Actual Outcomes. Introducing Lisa, the Fiber Addict Lisa suffered from addictions. She included the soluble fiber psyllium husk into her morning regimen. The outcome less binge eating and a consistent drop in weight.

Technical Assistance: Psyllium husk balances blood sugar levels and encourages fullness.

Insert Mark Here: The Magnesium Expert Mark's anxiety skyrocketed. He began supplementing with magnesium. His desires brought on by stress disappeared, and his sleep improved.

Expert Approval: Nutritionist Dr. Rodriguez extols the virtues of magnesium for reducing stress and promoting general health.

3. Expert Opinions. Endocrinologist Dr. Patel: While they might be useful tools, supplements are not quick fixes. Add these to attentive eating and exercise.

Nurse Emily's words of wisdom: Remember that vitamins complement the main course much as spices do. Don't depend on them alone.

Now that we have finished our investigation of supplements, let's move smoothly on to the next chapter, Lifelong Fitness. Your metamorphosis is waiting for you as the trip continues!

Chapter 6: Health in the Long Run

The Path to Enduring Health. Setting sail on the huge ocean of wellbeing is what it feels like to embark on a weight reduction journey. The real journey, however, is staying on track long after the first few pounds are gone. This chapter serves as a guide for you while you traverse the long-term health seas.

1. The Foundations of Long-Term Health

Consistency Over Intensity: The foundation of long-term health is made up of little, everyday routines. Your future is shaped by your constancy, not by the ferocity of your deeds.

Connectivity and Mindfulness: Pay attention to your body's cues. Encourage a relationship with food that is centered on nourishing rather than restricting it.

2. Health in Harmony

Equanimity in Everything: Your life has to be a harmonious combination of action, rest, and nourishment, much like a symphony does with different instruments.

The Tempo of Daily Life: Create a schedule that suits your way of living. Allow it to be both adaptable and sufficiently organized to help you achieve your objectives.

3. The Community Tapestry

Shared Journeys: Be in the company of others who encourage and support you in achieving your wellness objectives. You may create a tapestry of support and responsibility together.

Celebrating Milestones: Celebrate each accomplishment, no matter how little. Every one of them is a strand in the greater tapestry of your tale of well-being.

4. The Well-Being Wisely

Lifelong Learning: Continue to be inquisitive about wellbeing and health. Accept fresh information and be prepared to modify your strategy as you go.

Explaining By Example: Tell others about your trip. Your experience may help someone else find their way to wellness.

Recall that the quest for long-term well-being doesn't stop here as we complete this chapter. You are capable of handling this continuing journey with poise and resiliency. Get ready to flip to the next chapter, where we delve into Creating Long-Term Routines that will motivate and direct you towards a lifetime of well-being.

6.1 Creating Long-Term Routines

The Plan for Long-Term Transformation. Building strong habits is like building a bridge: it links your current behavior to your well-being in the future. Let's establish the groundwork for long-lasting behaviors.

1. The Foundations of Habit Development

Start Small, Think Big: Make small changes at first. Over the course of weeks and months, these apparently little deeds add up to determine your fate.

The Consistency Factor: Consider a leaking faucet: although it may not seem like much, each drop creates a groove in the rock. Reliability shapes your behaviors.

2. How to Stack Your Habits Connecting Moves: Add new routines to ones that already exist. Do you get your teeth brushed After, add a minute to stretch. It quickly becomes automatic.

Get to Know Jane: The Habit Designer: Busy professional Jane combined writing about thankfulness with her daily coffee regimen. Her days changed.

3. The Anchors of Emotion

Emotions Drive behaviors: Your emotions serve as the foundation for behaviors. You lace up your shoes with excitement as you think about joy and a morning stroll.

The Sunset Meditation: As you meditate, see the sun lowering. Soon, the arrival of twilight brings about serenity the completion of a habit cycle.

4. The Effect of Ripples. One Habit, Many Benefits: Habits cast ripples across life, much like a pebble placed into a pond. Exercise

improves mood and concentration in addition to increasing fitness.

Teaching By Example: Talk about how you developed your habit. You never know who else's metamorphosis you could inspire.

Now that we have finished our investigation of sustainable behaviors, let's move smoothly on to the next subchapter: The Importance of Sleep. Get ready to discover the keys to peaceful evenings and vibrant days.

6.2 The Significance of Rest

Welcoming the Night: The Function of Sleep. Sleep is the thread that connects our physical and mental well-being in the wellness tapestry. It is the unsung hero of our everyday lives, the quiet healer, and the invisible restorer.

1. Sleep: The Basis of Well-Being.

Rejuvenating Sleep: Every night when we go to sleep, our bodies start a process of renewal and healing. Hormone balance, muscles expand, and cells rejuvenate.

Emotional Balance: Sleep is the conductor of our mental symphony; it keeps our memory, concentration, and judgment in perfect harmony.

2. The Sleep-Wellness Connection

Immune Resilience: A rested body acts as a stronghold. Our immunity is strengthened by sleep, which protects us from disease.

Emotional Equilibrium: Getting enough sleep soothes the spirit, bringing about inner serenity and softening the edges of our emotions.

3. Sleep: A Chronicle

Stories of Metamorphosis: Take Anna, whose sleeplessness completely changed her life. Her nights and days were recaptured by her mindful sleep practices.

The Sleep Science: Sleeping for seven to nine hours a night may be the key to optimum health, according to studies.

4. Creating Your Dream Sleep Environment, The Environment Is Important: Make your bedroom a calm, dark, and peaceful sanctuary.

Make your bedroom a haven from the hectic outside world.

Rest Rituals: Create routines before going to bed. A book, a cup of herbal tea, or some light stretching might help your body know when it's time to relax.

With the closing of this chapter on sleep, let's get ready to move on to the next subchapter, Stress Management Techniques. There, we'll learn how to unleash the calm within and conquer the beast of stress.

6.3 Stress-Management Techniques

Navigating the Storm: Calming the Waves of Stress. Stress is the storm that rages inside us, threatening to capsize our wellness ship. But don't worry, we have tools to help us steady the ship and navigate life's tumultuous waves.

1. The Art of Mindfulness

Current Anchors: Mindfulness urges us to focus our attention on the present moment. Breathe. Feel the earth underneath your feet. Allow your troubles to float away.

Meet Alex, the Mindful Teacher: Alex, a frazzled teacher, found mindfulness after a hectic school day. One minute of concentrated breathing changed her classroom and her life.

2. The Power of Breathing

The Breath Bridge: Inhale bravery; expel stress. Your breathing is the link between chaos and tranquility.

The 4-7-8 Technique: Breathe in for four counts, hold for seven, then exhale for eight. Repeat. It is a lullaby for your nervous system.

3. Sanctuary Within

Visionary Retreats: Close your eyes. Consider a calm setting, such as a sun-drenched beach, a mossy woodland, or a comfortable library. Visit often.

The Stress Relief Playlist: Music comforts the soul. Make a playlist with relaxing songs. Let melodies untie your anxieties.

4. The Ripple Effect of Self-Care

Self-Care Rituals: Self-care is similar to gardening in that it takes daily attention. A warm bath, a cup of herbal tea, or a diary entry each drop promotes your overall well-being.

Example-Based Teaching Please share your self-care journey. Your ripple may inspire someone else's haven of peace.

As we wrap up our stress management discussion, let's move on to the following subchapter: Lifelong Fitness. We'll lace up our shoes and dance with health.

6.4 Lifelong Fitness.

The Symphony of Movement. Fitness is not a goal it is the rhythm that we follow throughout our lives. Let's look at how movement becomes a lifetime partner, bringing us strength, flexibility, and pleasure.

1. The Dance of Daily Activities. Every Step Counts: Whether it's a brisk stroll, a fun dance, or a yoga flow, movement is medicine. Most days, try to get in at least 30 minutes.

Meet Carlos, the Office Dancer: Carlos, a desk-bound accountant, realized the power of short breaks. Every hour, he swayed to his favorite song. His excitement increased, and his coworkers joined in the dancing.

2. Strength Ensemble. Muscles as allies: Strength training focuses on functional vitality rather than bulging biceps. Lift weights, use bodyweight workouts, or use resistance bands.

Graceful aging: Strong muscles help us age well by protecting our joints, maintaining balance, and improving our quality of life.

3. The Flexible Waltz. Supple Bodies, Supple Minds: Yoga, Pilates, and stretching help keep our bodies flexible. However, they also relax our thoughts, releasing tension knots.

The Sunset Stretch: Imagine stretching as the sun sinks under the horizon. Every elongation says, Release, renew.

4. The Beat of Cardio, Health of the Cardiovascular System: Our hearts are tireless drummers. Cardio exercises such as jogging, cycling, and swimming keep the heart rate stable.

• The Runner's High: Meet Maria, who discovered consolation in jogging. Her feet hammering the concrete symbolized her inner strength.

As we end our investigation of lifetime fitness, let us prepare for the next chapter: Transformation Stories. We'll meet real-life heroes who danced their way to health. Their stories will inspire and guide you on your own transformational path.

Chapter 7: Transformation Stories.

The Mosaic of Change. Every transformation tale is a work of art, a narrative that depicts the realm of potential. In this chapter, we tell the stories of people who have followed the road of health and emerged changed.

1. Tapestry of Triumph, Tales of Resilience: From the mother who juggled parenthood and exercise to the entrepreneur who found balance amid upheaval, their tales provide hope.

The Power of Perseverance: Each narrative emphasizes a universal truth: the unwavering strength of the human spirit.

2. Chronicles of Change. Journeys of Discovery: These aren't simply weight loss tales they're also about self-discovery, finding strength in vulnerability and bravery in adversity.

The Lessons Learned: Every tale contains valuable lessons, methods, and insights that you may use in your own lives.

3. The Ripple Effect of Wellness, Inspirational Action: These tales are meant to be experienced rather than just read. They will motivate you to start your own travels.

The Community for Change: As readers flip the pages, they become part of a community bound together by a common goal of healing.

4. Celebration of Transformation, Honoring Each Step: Every minor accomplishment is cherished, and every failure serves as a learning opportunity. The journey is as vital as the goal.

The Symphony of Success: These tales work together to build a symphony of success, a tune that speaks to the possibilities of change.

As we flip the page on these transformation tales, we take with us the melodies of change. They remind us that our own tale is ready to be written and that we may modify ourselves. Prepare to begin the next chapter, where we will investigate the Ripple Effect of Wellness. We'll explore how personal transformation may promote communal and global well-being.

7.1 Inspirational Journeys of Change

The strength of the human spirit a force that defies odds and rewrites destinies is essential to change. This subchapter is devoted to the brave people who have accepted change and emerged triumphant, not just physically but also in their whole view on life. Change often starts with a spark a moment of clarity when the need for change becomes obvious. Some people are concerned about their health, while others want to enjoy their lives to the utmost.

Embracing the challenge

First Steps: A thousand mile trip starts with one step. It's about committing to one day at a time.

The Support System: Nobody travels this route alone. Friends, family, and even strangers who share similar journeys become pillars of support.

Stories to Stir the Soul

The marathoner: Meet Michael, a former couch potato who now runs marathons. His secret One run at a time, propelled by the shouts of his loved ones.

A Mindful Eater: Sarah changed her connection with food by practicing mindfulness, learning to relish each meal, and paying attention to her body's requirements.

Lessons from the Road

Persistence versus Perfection: The path to transformation is paved with setbacks. Persistence, rather than perfection, is what generates long-term change.

Small Habits, Large Impact: Tiny behaviors may lead to major changes. Small, regular adjustments create a new reality.

Inspiration for Others: Each narrative is like a pebble tossed into the water of mankind, causing ripples that encourage others to go on their own path.

The Collective Movement: These tales are more than simply personal successes, they are part of a larger movement for a better, happier planet.

As we flip the page on these inspirational travels, we prepare to dive into the following subchapter, 7.2 Lessons Learned. Here, we shall extract the lessons learned from these events, providing a road map for those who dare to dream of change.

7.2 Lessons Learned

In the road of change, each tale is a chapter, and every chapter is packed with lessons. This subchapter is a treasure mine of information collected from the lived experiences of people who have traveled the road of healing and emerged enlightened. The Wisdom of Experience. The essential worth of transformation tales rests not simply in the results, but in the rich lessons they give. These teachings are beacons that illuminate the way for others on their road to well-being.

Embracing the Process

The Journey Matters: It's not only the destination but the trip that molds us. Embrace each step, each hardship, and each victory.

The Power of Adaptability: Be flexible in your approach. What works for one may not work for another. Adapt, learn, and develop.

Strategies for Success

Consistency is Key: The most prevalent thread in all tales of transformation is constancy. It's the everyday behaviors that establish a lifetime of well-being.

Mindset Shifts: A change of the body starts with a makeover of the mind. Cultivate a growth attitude that sees opportunities, not restrictions.

Overcoming Obstacles

Learning from Setbacks: Each problem is a chance to learn. When confronted with hurdles, seek for the lesson, not the loss.

Resilience and Recovery: The route to well-being is not linear. Learn to bounce back with more strength and knowledge.

The Collective Wisdom

Shared Knowledge: Transformation tales are not simply personal experiences, they are communal knowledge handed on to inspire and lead.

The Universal Lessons: These tales educate us about the universal elements of change discipline, patience, tenacity, and the power of community.

As we reflect on these lessons learned, we prepare to walk into the following subchapter, 7.3 The Ripple Effect of Wellness. Here, we will examine how personal development may unleash waves of good change in communities and beyond.

7.3 The Ripple Effect of Wellness

Creating Waves of Positive Change. Wellness isn't a single activity, it's a ripple that stretches well beyond our own lives. In this subchapter, we investigate how personal development may produce a tidal wave of well-being, reaching communities, families, and even the planet.

1. The Butterfly Effect, Small Actions, Big Impact: Imagine a butterfly waving its wings a seemingly minor action. Yet, it sets off a chain reaction that resonates across countries. Our healthy choices are like those butterfly wings.

Inspiring Others: When we emphasize health, we encourage people around us. Our children, friends, and coworkers watch our routines and learn from our example.

2. The Community Connection, The Power of Collective Wellness: A healthy community

flourishes together. It's not only about individual health, it's about establishing surroundings that foster well-being.

Local Initiatives: From community gardens to fitness programs, local initiatives produce a rippling effect. When one person joins, others follow.

3. The Global Web of Wellness, A World in Balance: Imagine if every individual made tiny changes choosing stairs over elevators, opting for healthy meals, practicing mindfulness. The combined effect would be significant.

Global Movements: Social media links us internationally. Wellness challenges, virtual walks, and shared recipes build a network of well-being that transcends boundaries.

4. The Legacy We Leave

Planting Seeds: Our deeds now sow seeds for future generations. When we emphasize well-being, we leave a legacy of health awareness.

The Echo of Inspiration: Our tales encourage others to begin on their own health journeys. Each altered life becomes a beacon for change.

As we end our investigation of the ripple effect, let's be ready to walk into the following subchapter: 7.4 Lifelong Learning. Here, we'll dig into the art of ongoing development and the thrill of lifetime discovery.

7.4 Maintaining Your Transformation

The Art of Sustaining Change, The path to health is not a sprint, it's a marathon a constant commitment to the ideas that have brought you to where you are today. This subchapter is devoted to the skill of preserving the change you've worked so hard to create.

1. The Pillars of Sustained Success

Consistent Routines: The key to preserving your change is consistency. Establish routines that blend easily into your life.

Mindful Awareness: Stay tuned with your body's cues. Mindfulness keeps you alert to your requirements and helps avoid old behaviors from coming back.

2. Case Studies: Stories of Enduring Change

The Resilient Spirit: Meet James, who dropped 50 pounds and has kept it off for five years. His secret, A balanced diet and frequent exercise, accompanied by a strong network of friends.

The Lifelong Learner: Lisa accepted knowledge as her instrument. She learned about nutrition and exercise, which allowed her to make educated decisions every day.

3. Scientific Backing: The Evidence of Effectiveness

Research Revelations: Studies demonstrate that behavioral therapies may lead to sustained weight reduction, particularly when accompanied by assistance from healthcare professionals.

Professional Endorsements: Healthcare specialists advise a comprehensive approach to weight control, stressing the significance of lifestyle changes over short fixes.

4. Testimonials: Voices of Validation

The Healthcare Champion: Sustainable weight reduction is feasible via consistent work and lifestyle modifications. It's about making better choices every day, comments Dr. Smith, a recognized nutritionist.

The Fitness Advocate: Transformation is not merely physical. It's a mental and emotional journey that demands support and self-compassion, adds Emily, a fitness coach.

Conclusion: The Journey Continues

As we end this chapter, remember that sustaining your change is a continual process. It's about growing with your changing needs and circumstances, and continuously aiming for balance and wellbeing.

www.ingramcontent.com/pod-product-compliance
Lightning Source LLC
Chambersburg PA
CBHW051834250726
48659CB00005B/1833